KALE
The Nutritional *Powerhouse*

Beverly Lynn Bennett

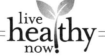

HEALTHY LIVING PUBLICATIONS
Summertown, Tennessee

Cover and interior design: Scattaregia Design

Healthy Living Publications,
a division of Book Publishing Company
P.O. Box 99
Summertown, TN 38483
888-260-8458
bookpubco.com

ISBN 978-1-57067-325-2

20 19 18 17 16 15   1 2 3 4 5 6 7 8 9

Library of Congress Cataloging-in-Publication Data

Bennett, Beverly Lynn.
  Kale : the nutritional powerhouse / Beverly Lynn Bennett.
    pages cm
  Includes index.
  ISBN 978-1-57067-325-2 (pbk.) -- ISBN 978-1-57067-874-5 (ebook)
  1. Cooking (Kale) 2. Kale. 3. Nutrition. I. Title.
  TX803.G74B46 2015
  641.6'5347--dc23
                  2014046260

Printed on recycled paper

Book Publishing Company is a member of Green Press Initiative. We chose to print this title on paper with 100% post-consumer recycled content, processed without chlorine, which saved the following natural resources:

- 18 trees
- 563 pounds of solid waste
- 8,414 gallons of water
- 1,551 pounds of greenhouse gases
- 8 million BTU of energy

BOOK PUBLISHING CO.

green press INITIATIVE

For more information on Green Press Initiative, visit www.greenpressinitiative.org. Environmental impact estimates were made using the Environmental Defense Fund Paper Calculator. For more information, visit papercalculator.org.

CONTENTS

Acknowledgments

I'd like to thank several people for their support and assistance during the writing of this book: fellow kale devotees, Cynthia and Bob Holzapfel and Jo Stepaniak, for their encouragement and guidance during the writing and editing processes involved with making this book a reality. My husband, Ray Sammartano, for his enduring love for me and what I do, for his invaluable tech support and insightful comments, and especially for eating tons of kale with me as my chief taste tester during the recipe-development process. Luna, my feline companion, for supervising me in the kitchen while I was creating the recipes and for the many purring sessions on my lap when I needed a break from writing. My family, for all of their encouraging words and loving support, and the farmers of the Eugene, Oregon, area for growing all the fabulous, organic kale that I used in creating the recipes for this book. Last but not least, all the vegans in the world for choosing to improve their lives, the lives of animals, and the future of this planet. Thank you for living with awareness and making a difference.

Introduction

Many nutrition experts consider kale among the top ten vegetables that we should include in our diets. This highly praised member of the plant kingdom is so well admired that it's often referred to as "King Kale" or the "Queen of Greens" by health aficionados and kale devotees. Kale is a member of the brassica family, which includes cruciferous vegetables, such as broccoli, Brussels sprouts, cabbage, cauliflower, collard greens, kale, kohlrabi, and turnips. More commonly, kale is classified as a dark leafy green, even though it comes in a wide variety of textures and colors, including assorted shades of green, purple, red, and white. Unlike cabbage, kale doesn't form a head. Instead, the leaves sprout from a central stalk, although some kinds grow in small clumps of individual leaves.

In the last decade, kale has become quite trendy, as health-conscious people are making a concerted effort to include more of it in their meals. To keep up with the current kale craze, grocery stores are stocking more varieties of kale and kale-based products, such as the widely popular crispy kale chips. Kale-spiked green juices and smoothies are making an appearance at most juice bars, and restaurants from coast to coast are adding more kale dishes to their menus, including kale salads, kale-enhanced soups and stews, and braised kale. Although kale may seem like just another culinary fad or the latest food sensation, it's in fact one the oldest cultivated vegetables.

Nutritional Benefits of Kale

In recent years, the term "superfood" has been increasingly used to describe certain fruits and vegetables. While there is no scientific definition of the word "superfood," most health authorities agree that in order for a food to be labeled as such, it should contain higher than usual amounts of vitamins, minerals, and other vital nutrients. Kale most definitely belongs in the superfood category, as its nutrient profile is quite impressive. Eating kale not only provides a lengthy list of nutritional benefits, but it also has been deemed capable of preventing and combating many health issues, chronic illnesses, and diseases.

Kale is an excellent source of several essential vitamins, including A, C, E, K, and various B vitamins. It's also a rich source of many minerals, such as calcium, copper, magnesium, manganese, phosphorus, potassium, and iron. Furthermore, kale is alkalizing; it can lessen the body's need for acid-neutralizing minerals, such as calcium, magnesium, and potassium, which the body uses to maintain proper mineral and pH balance. Vegans and others who avoid dairy products are often questioned about where they get their calcium. The answer is easy! Simply eating plenty of kale provides a megadose of calcium in an easily assimilated form that can actually decrease the body's requirement for calcium. Score one for the plant kingdom!

Additionally, vegans and vegetarians will be happy to know that kale is an amazing source of plant-based protein. In fact, just like many kinds of meat, kale contains all nine essential amino acids, which the body needs to form proteins. But that's not all. Kale also contains nine other nonessential amino acids. That's pretty impressive for a humble leafy green vegetable!

Moreover, kale is an excellent source of alpha-linolenic acid (ALA), an omega-3 fatty acid that is essential for brain health, boosts heart health, and decreases the risk of developing type2 diabetes. Plus, kale is low in calories, fat, and carbohydrates while being high in dietary fiber. All of these attributes can aid in weight management. The fiber contained in kale also helps to bind bile acids, assists in digestion and elimination, regulates blood sugar, and lowers cholesterol levels, which in turn can reduce the risk of developing diabetes and heart disease.

Nutritional Content of 1 Cup (250 ml) Raw Kale

calories: 33
carbohydrates: 7g
protein: 2 g
fat: 0.3 g
fiber: 1 g
omega-3 fatty acids: 121 mg
omega-6 fatty acids: 92 g

Source: United States Department of Agriculture, http://ndb.nal.usda.gov

Percent Daily Value of 1 Cup (250 ml) Raw Kale

vitamin K: 684%
vitamin A: 206%
vitamin C: 134%
manganese: 26%
copper: 10%
calcium and potassium: 9%
iron and magnesium: 6%
selenium, sodium, and zinc: trace amounts

Sources: nutritiondata.self.com; nationalkaleday.org; tracker.dailyburn.com

Kale is also a phenomenal source of antioxidants, which help to neutralize free radicals in the body and mitigate oxidative stress (caused by compromised oxygen metabolism) and chronic inflammation. Studies have shown that these conditions may be risk factors for myriad diseases. By simply increasing your kale consumption, you can also lower your risk of developing various types of cancers, such as bladder, breast, colon, ovarian, and prostate cancers.

In addition, kale contains dozens of different carotenoids and flavonoids, both of which have antioxidant and anti-inflammatory properties. Three carotenoids found in kale in significant amounts are beta-carotene, lutein, and zeaxanthin. Studies have shown that an increased consumption of carotenoid-rich fruits and vegetables helps to reduce the risk of age-related macular degeneration and cataracts, atherosclerosis, and chronic obstructive pulmonary disease. Two of the most notable flavonoids found in kale are kaempferol and quercetin, which not only have anti-inflammatory properties but also help to prevent arterial plaque formation.

Like other cruciferous vegetables, kale is a rich source of the sulfur-containing compounds known as glucosinolates, which contribute to the strong aroma and flavor associated with these types of vegetables. Chopping, chewing, or cooking kale helps to break down these glucosinolates and form other beneficial phytochemical by-products, such as indole-3 carbinol, isothiocyanates, and sulforaphane. While glucosinolates may not sound appealing from a taste standpoint, they are quite nutritionally beneficial, as studies have shown that they help to block the growth of cancer cells and assist in the detoxification processes of cells and organs.

Eating kale with citrus fruits or acidic foods makes the iron in kale more bioavailable. Similarly, when kale is cooked or served with fats, such as oil, avocado, nuts, or seeds, the fat-soluble carotenoids in the vegetable become more bioavailable. Strive to eat 1½ to 2 cups (375 ml to 500 ml) of kale several times a week so you can fortify your body with all these amazing nutritional benefits.

Cautionary Advice

While kale is indeed a nutritional powerhouse, people with certain health issues should heed a few precautions. If you suffer from digestive issues, be aware that for some people, eating raw kale can cause gas, bloating, abdominal pain, or other types of digestive distress. The good news is that cooking kale greatly reduces its gas-producing qualities.

Kale contains high levels of vitamin K, which plays a vital role in regulating blood clotting. If you take anticoagulant drugs, however, you should consult with your doctor to determine how often you should eat kale and what amounts are appropriate for you.

As with several other types of leafy greens, kale contains oxalates, which are naturally occurring acids that are found in plants, animals, and humans. Oxalates can greatly affect the body's absorption of calcium, iron, and magnesium. A buildup of oxalates in the body has the potential to cause functional problems for the gallbladder, kidneys, and thyroid; kidney stones or gallstones; and muscle pain or weakness. There is much dissension among health experts as to whether or not kale should be considered a low- or high-oxalate food, as the exact oxalate content of kale can vary greatly depending on the variety and whether it's being consumed raw or cooked (and how long it's been cooked). Therefore, check with your doctor if you have or experience any of these health problems.

People who suffer from thyroid disease may need to regulate their kale consumption, as kale contains compounds called goitrogens, which can reduce the body's ability to absorb iodine and suppress thyroid function. If you suffer from hypothyroidism, limit the amount of raw kale that you eat and instead opt for eating braised, boiled, steamed, or stewed kale, since cooking kale greatly decreases the concentration of these compounds.

Varieties of Kale

There are several types of kale, each with a slightly different flavor, texture, and color. I encourage you to try each type to discover which ones you prefer. The following list briefly describes each of the five main varieties of kale:

Curly kale. The most popular and most commonly available type of kale is green curly kale. It has tightly curled, slightly ruffled, crunchy, dense leaves with pale veins and thick stems that range from bright to dusty green, depending on the maturity of the leaves. Younger leaves tend to have a mild, slightly peppery flavor, and more mature leaves tend to be stronger or bitter tasting. This type of kale is also available in red and purple varieties, which are great for adding more color to dishes. Curly kale is excellent in raw dishes, salads, juices, and smoothies.

Russian kale. Russian kale, also known as Siberian kale, is an old European variety that was brought by Russian traders to Canada and then to the United States. It has long stems and large, smooth, flat green leaves with slightly fringed edges that resemble oak leaves. Its mild, slightly sweet and peppery flavor makes it great for use in salads, soups, and quick-cooking dishes. Russian kale is also available in red and purple varieties.

Tuscan kale. Tuscan kale goes by a wide range of different names: black cabbage, black kale, cavolo nero, dino kale, dinosaur kale, lacinato kale, nero di Toscano, Toscana kale, and Tuscan black palm kale. Tuscan kale is the favored variety grown in Italy and is often used in Italian and

European cuisine. It has very dark, bluish-green to almost-black leaves, which are narrow and spear-like, with smooth edges and deep grooves that resemble scales (hence the dinosaur nickname) and thick, flat stems.

Tuscan kale leaves fan out around a center base stalk like a palm tree. The extremely firm texture of Tuscan kale makes it an excellent choice in soups or stews, stir-fried dishes, or cooked dishes paired with beans, pasta, or polenta.

Kale raab. Also known as kale rabe, this type of kale is basically the tiny, yellow-flowering bud clusters and stems of kale. It appears in the spring, after the kale plant has survived through the long, cold winter. The plant is at the end of its life cycle and has begun to bolt (go to seed) in order to self-sow the next generation of kale. Kale raab is quite tender and has a slightly sweet flavor compared to mature kale. It's typically eaten cooked as whole spears or cut into bite-sized pieces. Kale raab tastes best when boiled, steamed, or stir-fried, alone or with other ingredients. It's also great in soups, stews, and other cooked dishes made with pasta or grains.

Flowering kale. Also known as ornamental kale or salad savoy, flowering kale is actually a misnomer, as it isn't known for its flowers but rather for the beauty of its decorative leaves. It comes in a wide range of colors, including white, light yellow, light to medium green, pink, deep rose, lavender, mauve, purple, and violet-blue, as well as variegated combinations of these colors. Flowering kale is frequently used in landscaping, in garden beds or containers, for adding decorative accents and borders; it's commonly planted around porches, patios, and walkways. This type of kale tolerates cold temperatures well and retains its vivid colors from fall through spring. Most flowering kale varieties are also edible. The leaves are generally more tender and milder in flavor, and the stems are less tough and fibrous than those of other kale varieties typically used in the kitchen. Flowering kale is often used in blends of mixed greens, by restaurants to garnish plates, and in salad bars to decoratively line and fill in the empty spaces between containers.

Shopping, Using, and Storing Tips

Nowadays, you can find kale in many different forms, usually sold by the bunch, at your local supermarket or natural food store. When shopping for fresh kale, look for leaves that are vibrant in color, crisp in texture, and free of spots or browned edges. Avoid kale that is limp or wilted or has yellow or blue leaves, veins, or stems (depending on the variety), or that has a strong cabbage-like odor.

Many stores offer washed and coarsely chopped fresh kale in the bagged salad section. Also, packages of frozen chopped kale can be found alongside frozen spinach in the freezer aisle. If you're trying to stretch your food budget further, shop for kale at your local farmers' market. You'll find the best prices there; plus, it's hard to beat the quality and flavor of produce purchased within hours of harvesting. I highly recommend buying organic kale whenever possible, as I think the flavor is far superior to that of conventionally grown kale, and it's always wise to minimize your exposure to pesticide residues.

Store fresh kale in the refrigerator; it should stay fresh for up to a week. However, the longer it's stored, the more bitter it may become. If you buy kale by the bunch, remove the rubber band or twisttie after you get it home, and store it loosely covered in a plastic or mesh storage bag or in a container with the lid slightly ajar. Keep it either in the crisper drawer or on the bottom shelf of the refrigerator. Hold off on washing fresh kale until you're ready to use it. Alternatively, you can wash it in advance as long as you spin it dry with a salad spinner or allow it to air-dry on a clean towel. A little moisture on the kale will keep it from wilting too quickly in the fridge, but excess moisture on the leaves will accelerate spoilage and could lead to slimy or soggy leaves.

Cleaning Kale

Kale, like other leafy greens, is commonly grown in fine, sandy soil. Rain and watering typically leave deposits of dirt, sand, and other grit clinging to the crevices of the leaves. To remove grit on kale, carefully and thoroughly rinse each kale leaf under cold running water and then put it in a colander to drain. Alternatively, put the kale leaves (with or without the stems) in a colander and vigorously rinse and toss them under cold running water several times.

I prefer to use the triple-washing technique, which is a cleaning procedure common to the food service and food processing industries. This is done by submerging the kale leaves (with or without the stems) in a very large bowl filled with cold water, swishing the leaves around a bit to help loosen any clinging dirt, and letting the leaves soak for a few minutes, which allows the dirt to sink to the bottom of the bowl. Then the kale is lifted out of the water and transferred to a colander to drain. I generally repeat the entire process two more times or until I don't see any dirt in the bottom of the bowl.

There is nothing more unnerving than taking the first bite of a kale dish and feeling the slight crunch of grit between your teeth. So whichever cleaning approach you prefer, make sure to thoroughly wash kale before using it. If you're using kale to make salads or kale chips, a salad spinner (or patting the kale dry with a towel) will help remove any excess water from the leaves.

Removing Kale Stems

The stems of kale leaves can be quite tough and fibrous, which is why most recipes call for leaves that have been stemmed. However, for dishes that are cooked a long time, such as soups and stews, you can keep the stems intact and thinly slice the leaves crosswise into strips.

There are two methods you can use for removing kale stems. For the knife method, put the kale leaf flat on a cutting board and make a long slice with a sharp knife on both sides of the center stem, as close to the stem as possible, running from the tip to the base of the leaf. For the hand method, simply turn the kale leaf upside down, hold it by the stem in one hand, fold the leaf in half lengthwise with the other hand, and starting at the base of the stem, pull downward along the stem to strip off the leafy portion.

If you want to stem kale leaves but would like to use the stems for another dish, just finely slice or chop the stems before adding them to soups, stir-fries, or casseroles.

Using Kale in Recipes

I've included both volume and weight measurements for kale in the following recipes, as the exact amount of kale needed may fluctuate depending on the variety used. Although the size of a bunch can vary slightly depending on the grower and supplier, an average bunch of kale contains eight to ten leaves and weighs around 1 pound/450 g (with stems). This is the standard I've used for the recipes in this book. Like most other types of leafy greens, kale reduces greatly in volume when cooked. One pound (450 g) of stemmed raw kale will yield between 5 and 6 cups (1.25 to 1.5 L) of leaves (lightly packed). The same amount after cooking will yield 1½ to 2 cups (375 to 500 ml), or enough for two to three servings.

Many chefs will often add a splash of vinegar or a squeeze of lemon (or other citrus) to heighten the flavors of a dish, especially when it contains strong or intensely flavored ingredients, such as kale, leafy greens, or other cruciferous vegetables. This added acidity can mellow, sweeten, and soften the flavor and texture of kale all at the same time.

Now that you know a lot about kale and how to clean, prepare, and store it, I hope that this information and the recipes that follow inspire you to include more kale in your daily diet. Get ready to be amazed by how easy it can be to incorporate kale into breakfast, lunch, and dinner dishes, as well as snacks, baked goods, and sweet treats. In doing so, you too will become a self-professed kale lover and proudly chant "All hail to the kale!"

Breakfast and Brunch Ideas

Glowing Green Smoothie   *Yield: 3 cups (750 ml), 2 servings*

Green smoothies got their moniker from the handful or so of leafy greens that's blended with the other smoothie ingredients, creating a beautiful green tint. They've become quite popular in recent years. This one is made with bananas, grapes, and your choice of other sweet fruit, plus an ample amount of kale, chia seeds, and fresh ginger, which not only revs up the flavor but also amps up your energy.

> 1 large fresh or frozen banana, broken into 3 pieces
> 1 cup (250 ml) fresh or frozen chopped sweet fruit (such as mango, melon, nectarine, peach, or pineapple)
> ½ cup (125 ml) seedless grapes
> 1½ cups (375 ml) stemmed and finely torn curly or Tuscan kale, lightly packed
> 2 cups (500 ml) coconut milk beverage or almond milk
> 1 tablespoon (15 ml) chia seeds
> 2 slices (¼ inch/5 mm thick) fresh ginger (peeling optional)
> ¾ cup (185 ml) ice cubes (optional)

Put all the ingredients in a blender in the order listed and process until completely smooth, 2 to 3 minutes. Stored in a sealed container, Glowing Green Smoothie will keep for 2 to 3 days in the refrigerator or 3 months in the freezer.

Per serving: 242 calories, 5 g protein, 8 g fat (5 g sat), 45 g carbohydrates, 25 mg sodium, 185 mg calcium, 9 g fiber

Blushing Berry Smoothie: Replace the sweet fruit with 1 cup (250 ml) of fresh or frozen berries and replace the green kale with red or purple curly or Russian kale.

Tofu and Kale Scramble
Yield: 4 cups (1 L)

In this eye-appealing recipe, a blend of spices is used to not only infuse tofu with great flavor but also give it a yellow tint reminiscent of scrambled eggs. The colorful hue plays nicely off the vibrant green of the fresh kale.

1 pound (450 g) firm or extra-firm tofu

2 tablespoons (30 ml) nutritional yeast flakes

1 tablespoon (15 ml) reduced-sodium tamari

1 teaspoon (5 ml) curry powder

1 teaspoon (5 ml) onion powder

½ teaspoon (2 ml) chili powder

2 teaspoons (10 ml) olive oil or other oil

⅔ cup (160 ml) diced yellow or red onion

4 cups (1 L) stemmed and very thinly sliced kale (any variety),
lightly packed

1½ tablespoons (22 ml) minced garlic

Sea salt

Freshly ground black pepper

Crumble the tofu into a medium bowl using your fingers. Add the nutritional yeast, tamari, curry powder, onion powder, and chili powder and stir well to evenly coat the tofu.

Put the oil and onion and in a large cast-iron or nonstick skillet and cook over medium-high heat, stirring occasionally, for 3 minutes. Add the tofu and cook, stirring occasionally, for 3 minutes. Add the kale and garlic, cover, and cook, stirring occasionally, until the kale is tender, 3 to 5 minutes. Season with salt and pepper to taste. Serve immediately.

Per 1 cup (250 ml): 266 calories, 23 g protein, 15 g fat (3 g sat), 12 g carbohydrates, 209 mg sodium, 194 mg calcium, 2 g fiber

Note: Analysis doesn't include sea salt or freshly ground black pepper to taste.

Sweet Potato and Kale Hash

Yield: 6 cups (1.5 L)

Using sweet potatoes instead of the average spud, along with some kale, red onion, and red bell pepper, enhances both the nutritional value and visual appeal of this breakfast hash.

2 large sweet potatoes, scrubbed (peeling optional) and cut into
½-inch (1 cm) cubes

1½ tablespoons (22 ml) olive oil or other oil

1 red onion, diced

1 red or orange bell pepper, diced

3 cups (750 ml) stemmed and very thinly sliced kale (any variety),
lightly packed

1½ tablespoons (22 ml) minced garlic

1 teaspoon (5 ml) dried oregano or thyme

1 teaspoon (5 ml) chili powder

½ teaspoon (2 ml) ground cumin

½ teaspoon (2 ml) ground coriander

½ teaspoon (2 ml) smoked paprika, or ¼ teaspoon (1 ml) chipotle
chile powder

¼ cup (60 ml) chopped fresh parsley or cilantro, lightly packed

1½ tablespoons (22 ml) nutritional yeast flakes

Sea salt

Freshly ground black pepper

Put the sweet potatoes and oil in a large cast-iron or nonstick skillet and cook over medium-high heat, stirring occasionally, for 5 minutes. Add the onion and bell pepper and cook, stirring occasionally, for 5 minutes.

Add the kale, garlic, oregano, chili powder, cumin, coriander, and smoked paprika and cook, stirring occasionally, until the kale is wilted and the other vegetables are tender, 5 to 7 minutes. Stir in the parsley and nutritional yeast. Season with salt and pepper to taste. Serve hot.

Per 1 cup (250 ml): 103 calories, 3 g protein, 4 g fat (1 g sat), 15 g carbohydrates, 62 mg sodium, 7 mg calcium, 3 g fiber

Note: Analysis doesn't include sea salt or freshly ground black pepper to taste.

Thyme-Scented Kale and Cheddar Biscuits

Yield: 8 biscuits

Fresh thyme adds another dimension of flavor to these tender biscuits, which are streaked with kale and vegan cheddar cheese. They are a welcome addition to any breakfast and make a great accompaniment to soups or stews.

> 2½ cups (600 ml) stemmed and finely chopped kale (any variety), lightly packed
>
> 1 cup (250 ml) unsweetened plain soy milk or other nondairy milk
>
> 1 tablespoon (15 ml) cider vinegar
>
> 3 cups (750 ml) unbleached all-purpose flour or whole wheat pastry flour, plus more as needed
>
> 3 tablespoons (45 ml) aluminum-free baking powder
>
> 2 tablespoons (30 ml) chopped fresh thyme, or 2 teaspoons (10 ml) dried
>
> 1½ tablespoons (22 ml) unbleached cane sugar
>
> ½ teaspoon (2 ml) sea salt
>
> ¼ cup (60 ml) cold nonhydrogenated vegan margarine
>
> ½ cup (125 ml) shredded vegan cheddar cheese

Preheat the oven to 425 degrees F (220 degrees C). Line a baking sheet with parchment paper or a silicone baking mat.

Steam the kale until tender, 5 to 7 minutes. Remove from the heat. Let cool for 3 minutes.

Put the soy milk and vinegar in a small bowl and stir until well combined. Refrigerate for 10 minutes to thicken.

Put the flour, baking powder, thyme, sugar, and salt in a large bowl and stir until well combined. Using your fingers or a fork, work the margarine into the flour mixture until it resembles coarse crumbs. Add the milk mixture and gently stir to combine. Gently stir in the kale and cheese.

Transfer the dough to a floured work surface and sprinkle a little additional flour over the top. Using your hands, flatten the dough into a 1-inch-thick (2.5 cm) rectangle. Using a floured 2-inch (5 cm) biscuit cutter, cut the dough (without twisting the cutter) into 8 biscuits. Alternatively, cut the dough with a knife into 8 squares.

Put the biscuits on the prepared baking sheet, either touching, for soft-sided biscuits, or spaced 2 inches (5 cm) apart, for biscuits with lightly browned sides. Bake for 10 to 12 minutes, or until golden brown on the bottom. Serve hot, warm, or at room temperature. Stored in a sealed container at room temperature, Thyme-Scented Kale and Cheddar Biscuits will keep for 3 days.

Per biscuit: 280 calories, 7 g protein, 8 g fat (2 g sat), 43 g carbohydrates, 586 mg sodium, 252 mg calcium, 2 g fiber

Gluten-Free Thyme-Scented Kale and Cheddar Biscuits: Replace the unbleached all-purpose flour with a gluten-free baking mix and add ¾ teaspoon (4 ml) of xanthan gum.

Lunch Options

Curried Lentil-Kale Stew
Yield: 12 cups (3 L)

An earthy and aromatic blend of curry powder, cumin, thyme, and cayenne pairs perfectly with kale and brown lentils to create a full-flavored and hearty batch of stew.

7 cups (1.75 L) water or no-salt-added vegetable broth

1 pound (450 g) dried brown lentils, sorted and rinsed

1 yellow onion, diced

3 stalks celery, diced

2 tablespoons (30 ml) minced garlic

1 tablespoon (15 ml) curry powder

2 teaspoons (10 ml) dried thyme

1 teaspoon (5 ml) ground cumin

¼ teaspoon (1 ml) cayenne

1 bay leaf

1 bunch (1 pound/450 g) kale (any variety), stemmed and coarsely chopped

1½ tablespoons (22 ml) nutritional yeast flakes

¼ cup (60 ml) chopped fresh cilantro or parsley, lightly packed

Sea salt

Freshly ground black pepper

Put the water, lentils, onion, celery, garlic, curry powder, thyme, cumin, cayenne, and bay leaf in a large soup pot and bring to a boil over high heat. Cover, decrease the heat to low, and simmer for 30 minutes.

Add the kale and nutritional yeast, cover, and cook until the lentils and kale are tender, 15 to 20 minutes. Stir in the cilantro. Remove from the heat. Remove the bay leaf. Season with salt and pepper to taste. Serve hot.

Per 1 cup (250 ml): 252 calories, 17 g protein, 1 g fat (0.4 g sat), 45 g carbohydrates, 52 mg sodium, 66 mg calcium, 19 g fiber

Note: Analysis doesn't include sea salt or freshly ground black pepper to taste.

Caldo Verde Soup

Yield: 10 cups (2.5 L)

Caldo verde in Portuguese literally translates to "green broth," but it's so much more than that. Filled with hearty ingredients, it's essential for cool winter nights and perfect for serving with a loaf of crusty bread to dip into the rich broth.

1 yellow onion, diced

1 red bell pepper, diced

3 stalks celery, diced

1 tablespoon (15 ml) olive oil

2 vegan spicy sausage links, thinly sliced

2 tablespoons (30 ml) minced garlic

4 cups (1 L) no-salt-added vegetable broth

3 medium potatoes, scrubbed (peeling optional) and cut into 1-inch (2.5 cm) cubes

1 package (10 ounces/304 g) frozen kale, or ½ bunch (8 ounces/230 g) kale (any variety), stemmed and coarsely chopped

3 tablespoons (45 ml) nutritional yeast flakes

1 bay leaf

1 can (15-ounce/450 g) salt-free kidney beans or white beans, drained and rinsed

¼ cup (60 ml) chopped fresh parsley, lightly packed

1½ teaspoons (7 ml) crushed red pepper flakes

Sea salt

Freshly ground black pepper

Put the onion, bell pepper, celery, and oil in a large soup pot and cook over medium-high heat, stirring often, for 3 minutes to soften. Add the sausage and garlic and cook, stirring often, for 2 minutes.

Add the vegetable broth, potatoes, kale, nutritional yeast, and bay leaf and bring to a boil over high heat. Cover, decrease the heat to low, and simmer for 45 minutes. Add the beans, parsley, and red pepper flakes and simmer uncovered for 10 minutes. Remove from the heat. Remove the bay leaf. Season with salt and pepper to taste. Serve hot.

Per 1 cup (250 ml): 157 calories, 10 g protein, 4 g fat (0.4 g sat), 22 g carbohydrates, 274 mg sodium, 65 mg calcium, 6 g fiber

Note: Analysis doesn't include sea salt or freshly ground black pepper to taste.

Kale Yeah! Salad

Yield: 8 cups (2 L)

This eye-catching salad is made with a multicolored combination of red kale, rainbow chard, crisp veggies, edamame, toasted almonds, and coconut flakes, which are all tossed together in a zesty, teriyaki-flavored dressing.

Teriyaki Dressing (½ cup/125 ml)

2 tablespoons (30 ml) reduced-sodium tamari

2 tablespoons (30 ml) toasted sesame oil

Zest and juice of 1 lime (2 teaspoons/10 ml zest
    and 2 tablespoons/30 ml juice)

1½ tablespoons (22 ml) minced garlic

1½ tablespoons (22 ml) peeled and grated fresh ginger

1 tablespoon (15 ml) brown rice vinegar or cider vinegar

2 teaspoons (10 ml) agave nectar

¼ teaspoon (1 ml) dry mustard

¼ teaspoon (1 ml) crushed red pepper flakes

¼ teaspoon (1 ml) freshly ground black pepper

Salad

4 cups (1 L) stemmed and thinly sliced red curly kale, lightly packed

4 cups (1 L) stemmed and thinly sliced rainbow Swiss chard,
    lightly packed

1 cup (250 ml) shredded red cabbage

1 cup (250 ml) shredded carrots

2 large stalks celery, halved lengthwise and thinly sliced

½ red or orange bell pepper, diced

½ cup (125 ml) frozen shelled edamame or frozen peas, thawed

⅓ cup (85 ml) thinly sliced green onions

⅓ cup (85 ml) chopped fresh cilantro or parsley, lightly packed

⅓ cup (85 ml) toasted sliced almonds

⅓ cup (85 ml) toasted unsweetened coconut flakes

1 tablespoon (15 ml) raw sesame seeds or hemp seeds

To make the dressing, put all the dressing ingredients in a small bowl and whisk until well combined. Stored in a sealed container in the refrigerator, Teriyaki Dressing will keep for 7 days.

To make the salad, put the kale in a large bowl and drizzle 3 tablespoons (45 ml) of the dressing over it. Using your hands, vigorously massage the kale until it begins to wilt, about 2 minutes.

Add the Swiss chard, cabbage, carrots, celery, bell pepper, edamame, green onions, and cilantro and gently toss. Drizzle the remaining dressing over the kale mixture and gently toss to combine. Set aside for 10 minutes to allow the flavors to blend and the kale to wilt further. Just before serving, scatter the almonds, coconut flakes, and sesame seeds over the top as a garnish or gently stir them into the salad. Serve immediately.

Per 1 cup (250 ml): 148 calories, 5 g protein, 10 g fat (4 g sat), 13 g carbohydrates, 306 mg sodium, 82 mg calcium, 4 g fiber

Avocado, Tomato, and Kale Salad

Yield: 6 cups (1.5 L)

No oil is needed for this salad. Instead, diced avocado, nutritional yeast, and lime zest and juice are vigorously massaged into bite-sized pieces of kale to create a naturally creamy dressing. Additional diced avocado, tomatoes, and pumpkin seeds add a pop of color and a crunchy contrast.

> 1 bunch (1 pound/450 g) green or red curly kale, stemmed
>   and torn into bite-sized pieces
> 2 Hass avocados, diced
> Zest and juice of 2 limes (4 teaspoons/20 ml zest; ¼ cup/60 ml juice)
> 1½ teaspoons (7 ml) nutritional yeast flakes
> ¼ teaspoon (1 ml) sea salt, plus more as needed
> ¼ teaspoon (1 ml) freshly ground black pepper, plus more as needed
> 1 cup (250 ml) halved cherry tomatoes or diced tomatoes
> ⅓ cup (85 ml) raw or toasted pumpkin seeds

Put the kale, half the avocado, the lime zest and juice, and nutritional yeast, salt, and pepper in a large bowl. Using your hands, vigorously massage the kale mixture until the kale begins to wilt and takes on a slightly cooked texture, 3 to 5 minutes. Set aside for 15 minutes to allow the flavors to blend and the kale to wilt further.

Add the remaining avocado and tomatoes and gently toss. Taste and add more salt and pepper if desired. Scatter the pumpkin seeds over the top. Serve immediately.

Per 1 cup (250 ml): 279 calories, 6 g protein, 20 g fat (3 g sat), 23 g carbohydrates, 135 mg sodium, 51 mg calcium, 7 g fiber

Variation: Replace the lime zest and juice with the zest and juice of 1 large lemon.

Tomato and Kale Bruschetta   *Yield: 8 servings*

Transform humble slices of toasted bread into something extraordinary by rubbing them with fresh garlic and topping them with a mixture of cooked kale and tomatoes. Serve as an open-faced sandwich alongside soup or salad or enjoy as an appetizer or snack.

6 large cloves garlic, peeled

1 tablespoon (15 ml) olive oil

½ teaspoon (2 ml) crushed red pepper flakes

1 bunch (1 pound/450 g) kale (any variety), stemmed and thinly sliced

1 medium tomato or 2 Roma tomatoes, diced

1½ teaspoons (7 ml) nutritional yeast flakes

Sea salt

Freshly ground black pepper

8 thick slices Italian or other bread, toasted

Thinly slice 4 of the garlic cloves. Cut the remaining 2 cloves of garlic in half lengthwise and set aside. Put the sliced garlic, oil, and red pepper flakes in a large cast-iron or nonstick skillet and cook over medium-high heat, stirring occasionally, for 1 minute. Add the kale and tomato and cook, stirring occasionally, until the kale is tender, 3 to 4 minutes. Stir in the nutritional yeast. Season with salt and pepper to taste. Remove from the heat.

Rub the halved garlic cloves over one side of each slice of toasted bread. Evenly top with the kale mixture. Serve immediately.

Per serving: 140 calories, 6 g protein, 3 g fat (1 g sat), 24 g carbohydrates, 205 mg sodium, 95 mg calcium, 2 g fiber

   Note: Analysis doesn't include sea salt or freshly ground black pepper to taste.

Kale Raab Bruschetta: Replace the kale with 2 bunches (1 pound/450 g) kale raab, coarsely chopped, and omit the tomato.

Supper Selections

Kale Veggie Burgers

Yield: 6 burgers

A colorful combination of fresh veggies and kale forms the base of these tasty gluten-free burgers. Serve them on plates or burger buns or even in pita bread, topped with your favorite condiments.

3 tablespoons (45 ml) water

1½ teaspoons (7 ml) chia seeds, or 1 tablespoon (15 ml) ground flaxseeds

1½ cups (375 ml) coarsely chopped crimini or white button mushrooms

½ cup (125 ml) diced red or orange bell pepper

1 tablespoon (15 ml) olive oil or other oil, plus more as needed

1 package (10-ounces/304 g) frozen mixed vegetables (carrots, corn, green beans, and peas)

½ bunch (8 ounces/246 g) green kale (any variety), stemmed and coarsely chopped

1½ tablespoons (22 ml) minced garlic

2 teaspoons (10 ml) chili powder

2 teaspoons (10 ml) Italian seasoning blend, or 1 teaspoon (5 ml) dried basil, ½ teaspoon (2 ml) dried oregano, and ½ teaspoon (2 ml) dried thyme

1¼ cups (310 ml) chickpea flour

⅓ cup (85 ml) chopped fresh parsley, lightly packed

2 tablespoons (30 ml) nutritional yeast flakes

2 tablespoons (30 ml) raw tahini or other seed or nut butter

½ teaspoon (2 ml) sea salt

½ teaspoon (2 ml) freshly ground black pepper

Put the water and chia seeds in a small bowl and whisk until well combined. Set aside for 15 minutes to thicken. Whisk again to break up any clumps of chia seeds.

Put the mushrooms, bell pepper, and oil in a large cast-iron or nonstick skillet and cook over medium-high heat, stirring occasionally, for 3 minutes. Add the mixed vegetables and cook, stirring occasionally, for 5 minutes. Add the kale, garlic, 1 teaspoon (5 ml) of the chili powder, and 1 teaspoon (5 ml) of the Italian seasoning blend and cook, stirring occasionally, until the kale is tender, 3 to 5 minutes. Remove from the heat and let cool for 5 minutes.

Transfer the vegetable mixture to a medium bowl. Add the chia seed mixture, chickpea flour, parsley, nutritional yeast, tahini, salt, pepper, and the remaining teaspoons of chili powder and Italian seasoning blend. Stir until well combined.

Put a piece of parchment paper on a large cutting board or baking sheet. Using your hands, evenly divide the burger mixture into six equal portions on the parchment paper and flatten each portion into a patty. Refrigerate for at least 1 hour to let the patties firm up slightly.

Lightly oil a large cast-iron or nonstick skillet and heat over medium-high heat. When the skillet is hot, cook the burgers in batches until golden brown on both sides, 3 to 5 minutes per side. Add additional oil to the skillet as needed to prevent the burgers from sticking.

Per burger: 196 calories, 10 g protein, 7 g fat (1 g sat), 26 g carbohydrates, 81 mg sodium (268 mg sodium), 96 mg calcium, 7 g fiber

Variation: Replace the chickpea flour with whole wheat flour or other flour of choice.

Southern-Style Braised Greens

Yield: 5 cups (1.25 L)

When leafy greens are braised (cooked in a small amount of liquid) with onions, garlic, and a few other sweet and savory ingredients, the result is a batch of tender greens immersed in a flavorful broth, affectionately known in the South as pot liquor. The delicious pot liquor is often sopped up with bits of cornbread, bread, or biscuits, such as Thyme-Scented Kale and Cheddar Biscuits (page 18).

1 large yellow onion, diced

1 tablespoon (15 ml) olive oil or other oil

2½ tablespoons (37 ml) minced garlic

1 teaspoon (5 ml) crushed red pepper flakes

1½ cups (375 ml) water or no-salt-added vegetable broth

1 tablespoon (15 ml) cider vinegar

1 tablespoon (15 ml) blackstrap molasses

1 bunch (1 pound/450 g) kale (any variety), stemmed and thinly sliced

1 bunch (1 pound/450 g) leafy greens (such as collard greens, turnip greens, Swiss chard, or a combination), stemmed and thinly sliced

1½ tablespoons (22 ml) nutritional yeast flakes

Sea salt

Freshly ground black pepper

Hot sauce (optional)

Put the onion and oil in a large pot and cook over medium-high heat, stirring occasionally, for 5 minutes. Add the garlic and red pepper flakes and cook, stirring occasionally, for 1 minute.

Add the water, vinegar, and molasses and bring to a boil. Add the kale, cover, and cook until the kale begins to wilt, 2 to 3 minutes. Add the leafy greens, cover, and cook until the greens begin to wilt, 2 to 3 minutes. Stir, cover, decrease the heat to low, and simmer, stirring occasionally, until the kale and leafy greens are as tender as you like, 45 to 60 minutes. Remove from the heat and stir in the nutritional yeast. Season with salt, pepper, and hot sauce, if using, to taste. Serve hot.

Per 1 cup (250 ml): 127 calories, 7 g protein, 4 g fat (0.3 g sat), 20 g carbohydrates, 63 mg sodium, 348 mg calcium, 7 g fiber

Note: Analysis doesn't include sea salt, freshly ground black pepper, or hot sauce to taste.

Southern-Style Braised Greens and Beans: Add 1½ cups (375 ml) of salt-free cooked or canned black-eyed peas, red beans, or other beans, drained and rinsed.

Polenta with White Beans and Kale Raab

Yield: 6 cups (1.5 L)

When a member of the brassica family, such as kale, starts to bolt during the spring or winter months, the tender flowering stalks are called raab. Kale raab is not only edible but also delicious, particularly when it's cooked with white beans, onions, and garlic and served atop a batch of creamy polenta.

Polenta

4 cups (1 L) water

½ teaspoon (2 ml) sea salt

1 cup (250 ml) medium or coarse cornmeal

1 tablespoon (15 ml) nutritional yeast flakes

1½ teaspoons (7 ml) olive oil

Kale Raab Topping

⅔ cup (160 ml) diced yellow onion

1 tablespoon (15 ml) olive oil

2 bunches (1 pound/450 g) kale raab, coarsely chopped

1½ tablespoons (22 ml) minced garlic

½ teaspoon (2 ml) crushed red pepper flakes

1 can (15 ounces/450 g) salt-free cannellini beans or other
     white beans, drained and rinsed

½ cup (125 ml) chopped fresh basil, lightly packed

1 tablespoon (15 ml) nutritional yeast flakes

Sea salt

Freshly ground black pepper

To make the polenta, put the water and salt in a large saucepan and bring to a boil over high heat. Decrease the heat to medium. Slowly add the cornmeal, whisking constantly to prevent lumps, and cook until the mixture begins to boil again, 1 to 2 minutes.

Decrease the heat to low. Cover and cook, stirring every 10 minutes with a long-handled spoon, until the polenta is very thick and begins to pull away from the sides of the saucepan, 30 to 35 minutes. Add the nutritional yeast and oil and stir until well combined. Remove from the heat.

While the polenta is cooking, prepare the kale raab topping. Put the onion and oil in a large cast-iron or nonstick skillet and cook over medium-high heat, stirring occasionally, until the onion is soft and lightly browned, about 5 minutes. Add the kale raab, garlic, and red pepper flakes and cook, stirring occasionally, until the kale raab is crisp-tender, about 5 minutes.

Add the beans, basil, and nutritional yeast and stir until well combined. Remove from the heat. Season with salt and pepper to taste. Put the polenta on a large platter or divide into individual servings and top with the kale raab topping. Serve hot.

Per 1 cup (250 ml): 203 calories, 11 g protein, 5 g fat (1 g sat), 29 g carbohydrates, 290 mg sodium, 197 mg calcium, 8 g fiber

Note: Analysis doesn't include sea salt or freshly ground black pepper to taste.

Kale and Pumpkin Seed Pesto Pasta

Yield: 4 servings

Traditionally, pesto is a savory paste made with basil, garlic, pine nuts, and olive oil. This version takes some liberties with this basic formulation by supplementing some of the fresh basil with fresh kale and swapping out the pricey pine nuts with pumpkin seeds. Toss the finished pesto with your favorite cooked pasta for a fast and easy supper.

Kale and Pumpkin Seed Pesto (1 cup/250 ml)

¼ cup (60 ml) raw or toasted pumpkin seeds

2 large cloves garlic

2 cups (500 ml) stemmed and finely torn kale (any variety),
     lightly packed

1 cup (250 ml) fresh basil leaves, lightly packed

Zest and juice of 1 lemon (1½ to 2 tablespoons/22 to 30 ml zest;
     3 to 4 tablespoons/45 to 60 ml juice)

2½ tablespoons (37 ml) nutritional yeast flakes

2 tablespoons (30 ml) olive oil

½ teaspoon (2 ml) sea salt

¼ teaspoon (1 ml) freshly ground black pepper

Pasta

1 pound (450 g) spaghetti, fettuccine, penne, or rotini

Zest of 1 lemon (1½ to 2 tablespoons/22 to 30 ml zest)

Crushed red pepper flakes

To make the pesto, put the pumpkin seeds and garlic in a food processor and process until the pumpkin seeds are finely ground, about 1 minute. Add the kale, basil, lemon zest and juice, nutritional yeast, oil, salt, and pepper and process into a smooth paste, 1 to 2 minutes. Stored in a sealed container, Kale and Pumpkin Seed Pesto will keep for 5 to 7 days in the refrigerator or 3 months in the freezer.

To cook the pasta, fill a large pot two-thirds full with water and bring to a boil over medium-high heat. Add the pasta and cook, stirring occasionally, according to the package instructions or until the pasta is tender.

Using a ladle, transfer ½ cup (125 ml) of the pasta cooking water to a small bowl. Drain the pasta in a colander and return it to the pot. Depending on the pasta used, add ½ to 1 cup (125 to 250 ml) of the Kale and Pumpkin Seed Pesto and the reserved pasta cooking water to the cooked pasta and toss until evenly coated. Garnish with the lemon zest and red pepper flakes to taste. Serve hot.

Per serving: 537 calories, 19 g protein, 12 g fat (1 g sat), 92 g carbohydrates, 298 mg sodium, 104 mg calcium, 6 g fiber

Note: Analysis doesn't include crushed red pepper flakes to taste.

Colcannon

Yield: 7 cups (1.75 L)

One of the most well-known dishes of Celtic cuisine, colcannon could be simply described as enhanced mashed potatoes. Depending on the region where it's prepared, it traditionally consists of three basic components: potatoes; a member of the allium family, such as onion, leek, or green onion; and a vegetable from the brassica family, such as kale or cabbage.

3 pounds (1.4 kg) Yukon gold potatoes or other potatoes, peeled and cut into 2-inch (5 cm) cubes

1 leek, cut in half lengthwise, thoroughly rinsed, and thinly sliced

3 tablespoons (45 ml) nonhydrogenated vegan margarine

1 bunch (1 pound/450 g) kale (any variety), stemmed and very thinly sliced

1 cup (250 ml) soy milk or other nondairy milk

Sea salt

Freshly ground black or white pepper

Put the potatoes in a large pot, cover with water, and bring to a boil over high heat. Decrease the heat to low and simmer until the potatoes are soft, 15 to 20 minutes. Remove from the heat.

While the potatoes are cooking, put the leek and 1 tablespoon (15 ml) of the margarine in a large cast-iron or nonstick skillet and cook over medium-high heat, stirring occasionally, for 3 minutes. Add the kale and cook, stirring occasionally, until the kale is tender, 5 to 7 minutes. Remove from the heat.

Drain the potatoes in a colander and return them to the pot. Add the remaining 2 tablespoons (30 ml) of margarine and the soy milk. Using a potato masher, mash the mixture as smooth or chunky as desired. Add the kale mixture to the potatoes and stir until well combined. Season with salt and pepper to taste. Serve hot.

Per 1 cup (250 ml): 251 calories, 7 g protein, 6 g fat (2 g sat), 42 g carbohydrates, 93 mg sodium, 130 mg calcium, 7 g fiber

Note: Analysis doesn't include sea salt or freshly ground black pepper or white pepper to taste.

Snacks and Treats

Savory Kale Chips   *Yield: 6 cups (1.5 L)*

It's so easy to make a batch of crispy kale chips yourself, and homemade chips cost only a fraction of store-bought chips. In this recipe, a simple marinade and nutritional yeast are used to coat pieces of fresh kale to create one heck of a crunchy snack.

1 bunch (1 pound/450 g) curly or Tuscan kale, stemmed and torn into large bite-sized pieces

2 tablespoons (30 ml) nutritional yeast flakes

1½ tablespoons (22 ml) olive oil

1 tablespoon (15 ml) reduced-sodium tamari

1 teaspoon (5 ml) onion powder

1 teaspoon (5 ml) chili powder

1 teaspoon (5 ml) garlic powder

Using a salad spinner, thoroughly spin dry the kale in batches. Alternatively, use a clean towel or paper towels to completely pat dry the kale. Put the kale in a large bowl and set aside.

Put the nutritional yeast, oil, tamari, onion powder, chili powder, and garlic powder in a small bowl and whisk until well combined. Drizzle the oil mixture over the kale. Using your hands, gently massage the kale until it's evenly coated.

To dehydrate the kale chips, arrange the kale in a single layer on three or four dehydrator racks. Dehydrate until the kale is light and crispy, 4 to 6 hours. Alternatively, to bake the kale chips, see the baking instructions for Cheesy Kale Chips (page 37). Serve immediately.

Per 1 cup (250 ml): 72 calories, 3 g protein, 4 g fat (2 g sat), 9 g carbohydrates, 280 mg sodium, 108 mg calcium, 2 g fiber

Salt and Vinegar Kale Chips: Replace the tamari with 1½ tablespoons (22 ml) of vinegar (such as cider, balsamic, or sherry vinegar) and omit the nutritional yeast, chili powder, and garlic powder.

Cheesy Kale Chips

Yield: 6 cups (1.5 L)

A bell pepper and carrot are blended together with cashews, nutritional yeast, and a few other ingredients to create a creamy, cheesy sauce that is used to coat pieces of kale. After the kale is dehydrated or baked, it morphs into an indulgent-tasting snack.

1 bunch (1 pound/450 g) curly or Tuscan kale,
    stemmed and torn into large bite-sized pieces
¾ cup (185 ml) raw cashews, soaked in water for 1 hour and drained
1 red or orange bell pepper, diced
1 carrot, scrubbed (peeling optional) and diced
2 large cloves garlic
½ cup (125 ml) nutritional yeast flakes
Zest and juice of 1 lemon (1½ teaspoons/7 ml zest; ¼ cup/60 ml juice)
1 teaspoon (5 ml) agave nectar
1 teaspoon (5 ml) chili powder
1 teaspoon (5 ml) garlic powder
1 teaspoon (5 ml) ground turmeric
1 teaspoon (5 ml) sea salt

Using a salad spinner, thoroughly spin dry the kale in batches. Alternatively, use a clean towel or paper towels to completely pat dry the kale. Put the kale in a large bowl and set aside.

Put the cashews in a food processor and process until finely ground. Add the bell pepper, carrot, and garlic and process into a chunky purée, 1 to 2 minutes. Scrape down the sides of the container with a rubber spatula. Add the nutritional yeast, lemon zest and juice, agave nectar, chili powder, garlic powder, turmeric, and salt and process until smooth, 1 to 2 minutes. Pour over the kale. Using your hands, gently massage the kale until all the pieces are evenly coated.

To dehydrate the kale chips, arrange the kale in a single layer on three or four dehydrator racks. Dehydrate until the kale is light and crispy, 4 to 6 hours. Alternatively, to bake the kale chips, preheat the oven to 300 degrees F (180 degrees C). Line two large baking sheets with parchment paper or silicone baking mats. Arrange the kale in a single layer on the prepared baking sheets, dividing it equally between both sheets. Bake for 30 to 40 minutes, turning the kale over every 15 minutes, until it is light and crispy. Serve immediately.

Per 1 cup (250 ml): 156 calories, 10 g protein, 7 g fat (2 g sat), 20 g carbohydrates, 455 mg sodium, 119 mg calcium, 4 g fiber

Spicy Nacho Cheese Kale Chips: When processing the cashew mixture, add 1 jalapeño chile, seeded and finely diced. Add ½ teaspoon (2 ml) of smoked paprika and ½ teaspoon (2 ml) of cayenne or chipotle chile powder when processing the remaining cheese sauce ingredients.

Roasted Garlic and Kale Hummus

Yield: 2 cups (500 ml)

Here is a fresh take on the ever-popular Middle Eastern hummus that is flavored with roasted garlic and flecked with fresh kale and parsley. Enjoy this tasty combination as a dip with raw veggies, pita rounds, or crackers, or as a spread for sandwiches or wraps.

> 8 large cloves garlic, peeled
> 2 cups (500 ml) stemmed and finely chopped curly or Tuscan kale, lightly packed
> ½ cup (125 ml) fresh parsley, lightly packed
> Zest and juice of 1 lemon (1½ to 2 tablespoons/22 to 30 ml zest; 3 to 4 tablespoons/45 to 60 ml juice)
> 3 tablespoons (45 ml) water
> 1 can (15 ounces/450 g) salt-free chickpeas, drained and rinsed
> 3 tablespoons (45 ml) raw tahini
> 1½ tablespoons (22 ml) olive oil, plus more for garnish
> 1 teaspoon (5 ml) ground cumin, plus more for garnish
> ½ teaspoon (2 ml) sea salt
> Smoked or sweet paprika

Preheat the oven to 400 degrees F (200 degrees C).

Put the garlic on a piece of aluminum foil. Gather the corners of the foil, crimp to enclose the garlic, and put in a small baking pan. Bake for 20 to 30 minutes, or until the garlic is soft when gently squeezed.

Transfer the garlic to a food processor. Add the kale, parsley, lemon zest and juice, and water and process into a slightly chunky purée, 1 to 2 minutes. Scrape down the sides of the container with a rubber spatula. Add the chickpeas, tahini, oil, cumin, and salt and process until completely smooth, 1 to 2 minutes. Scrape down the sides of the container with a rubber spatula and process for 30 seconds longer.

Just before serving, drizzle with olive oil and sprinkle with cumin and paprika. Stored in a sealed container in the refrigerator, Roasted Garlic and Kale Hummus will keep for 5 to 7 days.

Per ¼ cup (60 ml): 104 calories, 4 g protein, 5 g fat (1 g sat), 13 g carbohydrates, 161 mg sodium, 73 mg calcium, 4 g fiber

Note: Analysis doesn't include smoked or sweet paprika or additional cumin or olive oil for garnish.

Hot Kale and Artichoke Dip

Yield: 8 servings

Spinach and artichoke dip gets a kale makeover. Prepared in a cast-iron skillet, this creamy dip is made with a savory mix of Tuscan kale, artichoke hearts, onions, and garlic, plus a lemon-accented vegan mozzarella cheese sauce. Serve it with thin slices of bread, melba toast, crackers, or crudités.

½ cup (125 ml) diced yellow onion

¼ cup (60 ml) olive oil

3 cups (750 ml) stemmed and finely chopped Tuscan kale, lightly packed

1½ tablespoons (22 ml) minced garlic

1 can (14 ounces/400 g) artichoke hearts packed in water, drained and coarsely chopped

2 cups (500 ml) soy milk or other nondairy milk

¼ cup (60 ml) nutritional yeast flakes

3 tablespoons (45 ml) tapioca starch

Zest and juice of 1 lemon (1½ to 2 tablespoons/22 to 30 ml zest; 3 to 4 tablespoons/45 to 60 ml juice)

1½ teaspoons (7 ml) Dijon mustard

1½ teaspoons (7 ml) dried basil

1 teaspoon (5 ml) sea salt

½ teaspoon (2 ml) crushed red pepper flakes

¼ teaspoon (1 ml) freshly ground black pepper

1 cup (250 ml) shredded vegan mozzarella cheese

Smoked or sweet paprika

Preheat the oven to 400 degrees F (200 degrees C).

Put the onion and 1½ teaspoons (7 ml) of the oil in a 10-inch (25 cm) cast-iron or other ovenproof skillet and cook over medium-high heat, stirring occasionally, for 3 minutes. Add the kale and garlic and cook, stirring occasionally, for 2 to 3 minutes, until the kale is tender. Stir in the artichoke hearts. Remove from the heat.

Put the soy milk, nutritional yeast, tapioca starch, lemon zest and juice, mustard, basil, salt, red pepper flakes, and pepper in a blender and process until completely smooth. Scrape down the sides of the jar with a rubber spatula and process for 30 seconds longer.

Add the soy milk mixture and cheese to the skillet and stir until well combined. Sprinkle the top with paprika. Bake for 25 to 30 minutes, until the dip is hot and bubbly around the edges. Serve hot.

Per serving: 101 calories, 4 g protein, 6 g fat (2 g sat), 10 g carbohydrates, 321 mg sodium, 36 mg calcium, 2 g fiber

Note: Analysis doesn't include smoked or sweet paprika for garnish.

Tip: To make 4 servings, cut the ingredient amounts in half and bake in an 8-inch (20 cm) skillet.

Double-Chocolate Kale Brownies

Yield: 9 brownies

Are you trying to get your family to eat more kale? Well, you'll definitely sneak one by them with this recipe, as melted chocolate chips and cocoa totally mask the flavor and color of the puréed kale that's been added to the batter of these rich and chewy vegan brownies.

2½ cups (600 ml) stemmed and coarsely chopped curly
     or Russian kale, lightly packed

2½ tablespoons (37 ml) water

1 cup (250 ml) unbleached sugar

½ cup (125 ml) unsweetened cacao powder or cocoa powder

¼ cup (60 ml) vegan chocolate chips, or 2 ounces (57 g) vegan
     chocolate, coarsely chopped

3 tablespoons (45 ml) nonhydrogenated vegan margarine

2 tablespoons (30 ml) chia seeds

1 teaspoon (5 ml) vanilla extract

¼ cup (60 ml) hot coffee or hot water

¾ cup (185 ml) unbleached all-purpose flour or
     whole wheat pastry flour

½ teaspoon (2 ml) sea salt

¼ teaspoon (1 ml) baking soda

Preheat oven to 350 degrees F (180 degrees C). Lightly oil an 8-inch (20 cm) square baking pan or mist it with cooking spray.

Steam the kale until soft and tender, 10 to 12 minutes. Remove from the heat. Set aside for 3 minutes to let the kale cool slightly. Transfer the kale to a food processor. Add the water and process for 1 minute. Scrape down the sides of the container with a rubber spatula and process until completely smooth, about 30 seconds longer.

Put the sugar, cacao powder, chocolate chips, margarine, chia seeds, and vanilla extract in a large bowl. Pour the hot coffee over the top, whisk until well combined, and set aside for 10 minutes. Whisk again to ensure that the chocolate chips and margarine are thoroughly melted and to break up any clumps of chia seeds.

Put the flour, salt, and baking soda in a small bowl and stir until well combined. Add the kale mixture to the chocolate mixture and whisk to combine. Add the flour mixture and whisk until well combined.

Transfer the batter to the prepared pan. Bake for 30 to 35 minutes, or until the center is set and a toothpick inserted in the center comes out clean. Let cool completely before cutting the brownies into squares. Stored in a lightly covered container at room temperature, Double-Chocolate Kale Brownies will keep for 3 days.

Per brownie: 215 calories, 4 g protein, 7 g fat (2 g sat), 35 g carbohydrates, 233 mg sodium, 27 mg calcium, 2 g fiber

Gluten-Free Double-Chocolate Kale Brownies: Replace the flour with a gluten-free baking mix and add ¼ teaspoon (1 ml) of xanthan gum.

Kale, Coconut, and Lime Cupcakes

Yield: 12 cupcakes

Blanching and shocking kale helps it retain its color and gives these cupcakes a vivid green hue. But it's the added coconut milk and fresh lime zest and juice that create their light texture and lusciously rich flavor. For a beautiful finish, the cupcakes are topped with a fluffy buttercream frosting and shredded coconut.

Cupcake Batter

3½ cups (875 ml) stemmed and finely torn curly or Russian kale,
    lightly packed

1½ cups (375 ml) coconut milk beverage

Zest and juice of 2 limes (4 teaspoons/20 ml zest; ¼ cup/60 ml juice)

3 tablespoons (45 ml) safflower oil or other oil of choice

1½ teaspoons (7 ml) vanilla extract

1½ cups (375 ml) unbleached all-purpose flour or
    whole wheat pastry flour

½ teaspoon (2 ml) aluminum-free baking powder

½ teaspoon (2 ml) baking soda

¼ teaspoon (1 ml) sea salt

Buttercream Frosting

⅓ cup (85 ml) nonhydrogenated vegan margarine

2½ cups (600 ml) powdered sugar

2 tablespoons (30 ml) coconut milk beverage

½ teaspoon (2 ml) vanilla extract

Unsweetened shredded dried coconut or coconut flakes

Preheat the oven to 375 degrees F (190 degrees C). Line a standard 12-cup muffin tin with paper or silicone liners, or lightly oil or mist it with cooking spray.

To prepare the kale, put it in a large saucepan, cover with water, and bring to a boil over medium-high heat. Fill a medium bowl half full with ice water. Cook the kale in boiling water for 3 minutes. Using a slotted spoon, quickly remove the kale from the boiling water and plunge it into the ice water to stop the cooking process. Set aside for 2 minutes.

To make the cupcake batter, using your hands, squeeze dry the kale and transfer it to a blender. Add the coconut milk beverage, lime zest and juice, oil, and vanilla extract and process until smooth and only small flecks of kale are visible. Scrape down the sides of the jar with a rubber spatula. Add the flour, baking powder, baking soda, and salt and process for 30 seconds longer.

Fill the prepared muffin cups using a ¼-cup (60 ml) ice-cream scoop or measuring cup. Bake for 18 to 20 minutes, or until a toothpick inserted in the center comes out clean. Remove from the oven. Let cool in the muffin tin for 10 minutes. Then transfer the cupcakes to a rack to cool completely.

To make the frosting, put the margarine in a large bowl and beat with an electric mixer or a stand mixer on medium speed for 1 minute. Add the powdered sugar, coconut milk beverage, and vanilla extract and beat until light and fluffy, 2 to 3 minutes.

Spread the frosting over the cooled cupcakes with a knife. Sprinkle a little shredded coconut over the top of each cupcake for a light coating. Alternatively, for a heavier coating of coconut, gently dip the frosted cupcakes into a bowl of shredded coconut or coconut flakes as desired. Stored in a sealed container at room temperature, Kale, Coconut, and Lime Cupcakes will keep for 2 to 3 days.

Per cupcake: 246 calories, 2 g protein, 9 g fat (2 g sat), 39 g carbohydrates, 166 mg sodium, 35 mg calcium, 1 g fiber

Note: Analysis doesn't include shredded dried coconut or coconut flakes for topping.

Kale, Coconut, and Lime Snack Cake: Pour the prepared batter into an oiled 9-inch (23 cm) round or square baking pan and bake for 20 to 25 minutes, or until a toothpick inserted in the center comes out clean.

ABOUT THE AUTHOR

Beverly Lynn Bennett is an experienced vegan chef and baker, writer, and animal advocate who is passionate about showing the world how easy, delicious, and healthful it is to live and eat as a vegan. A certified food-service operations manager, she earned her culinary arts degree in 1988 and gained much practical experience in the years that followed, working in and managing vegan and vegetarian restaurants and natural food stores.

Vegan since the early 1990s, Beverly is the author of *Vegan Bites: Recipes for Singles, Chia: Using the Ancient Superfood, The Complete Idiot's Guide to Vegan Slow Cooking, The Complete Idiot's Guide to Gluten-Free Vegan Cooking*, and others. Her work has appeared in many national and international print publications, on public television and DVDs, and all over the web. She has hosted The Vegan Chef website at VeganChef.com since 1999 and has been a regular columnist for *VegNews* magazine since 2002.

Beverly currently lives and works in the very vegan-friendly city of Eugene, Oregon, where her love of organic, healthy, and vibrant foods fuels a passion for developing innovative vegan recipes. Her work appeals to a wide assortment of tastes and provides enticing plant-based alternatives for people with various dietary restrictions. When she isn't hard at work in the kitchen, she can be found offering advice on all things vegan, frequenting local farmers' markets, and helping educate others on issues related to veganism and health through cooking demos and speaking engagements.

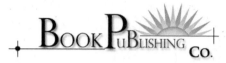

Book Publishing Co.

books that educate, inspire, and empower

A Holistic Approach to **ADHD** – *Deborah Merlin*

Weight Loss and Good Health with **APPLE CIDER VINEGAR** – *Cynthia Holzapfel*

Healthy and Beautiful with **COCONUT OIL** – *Cynthia Holzapfel and Laura Holzapfel*

The Weekend **DETOX** – *Jerry Lee Hutchens*

Enhance Your Health with **FERMENTED FOODS** – *Warren Jefferson*

Improve Digestion with **FOOD COMBINING** – *Steve Meyerowitz*

Understanding **GOUT** – *Warren Jefferson*

PALEO Smoothies – *Alan Roettinger*

Refreshing Fruit and Vegetable **SMOOTHIES** – *Robert Oser*

All titles in the **Live Healthy Now** series are only **$5.95!**

Interested in other health topics or healthy cookbooks?
See our complete line of titles at bookpubco.com or order
directly from:

Book Publishing Company
PO Box 99
Summertown, TN 38483
1-888-260-8458